IT COMES FROM WITHIN
Living with Bipolar Illness

MICHAEL SOLOMON
WITH GLORIA HOCHMAN

Philadelphia Daily News article page 65 reprinted with permission

Published 2018 by Shorehouse Books
Printed in the United States of America

Second Edition

ISBN-10: 0-9994127-7-9
ISBN-13: 978-0-9994127-7-0

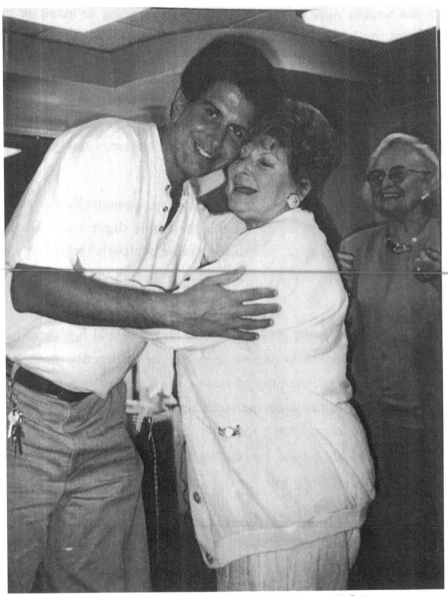

Mom was the Rainbow of my life!
Sylvia Dorothy Solomon
July 16, 1922 to January 30, 2006

For Abraham Martin Solomon and Sylvia Dorothy Solomon

and especially for Judy

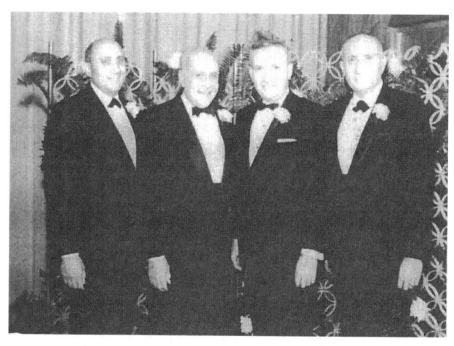

Left to right:
Uncle Mike – Uncle Mark – Uncle Max – Father Abraham Martin Solomon
The Four Solomon Brothers

Don't walk behind me; I may not lead. Don't walk in front of me; I may not follow. Just walk beside me and be my friend." -- Albert Camus

My dad Abraham Martin Solomon's favorite poem.

"My dad's business was AMS Food Brokerage and I would ask him what if your initials were ASS?" – Mike Solomon

Acknowledgements

The cover of this book was taken from a birthday card given to me by Dr. Barbara Granger, my former employer at Matrix Research Institute. The words she wrote to me, "Your Spirit Illuminates the World" represent the highest compliment I've ever received.

Rabbi Gary Charleston who has supported me emotionally. Thank G-d for the gift of his life.

Friend and neighbor Warren Levy who rescued me during a 2002 manic episode.

My team: my psychiatrist, William Packard; the caring staff at Penn Medicine, the kind people at Rosemont Pharmacy and my vocational counselor Don Helpa who recently retired and remains a good friend .

Kate Jackson, our family housekeeper, who was like a surrogate mother to me. She always introduced me as "my Michael."

CONTENTS

FOREWORD
Gloria Hochman 1

INTRODUCTION
My Friend Michael 3
Richard C. Baron

Hello, I'm Michael Solomon 5

ONE   What Is Bipolar Illness Anyway? 6

TWO   How Did I Get This Way? 8

THREE   Looking Backward 12

FOUR   A Rocky Road Ahead 16

FIVE   My Worst Manic Episode 18

SIX   My Dad Can't Die, Can He? 20

SEVEN   Life in Psychiatric Centers 22

EIGHT   Treatments That Transform 24

NINE   A New Start 30

TEN   The Power of Peers...The Miracle of Friendship 33

ELEVEN Spreading the Word 35

TWELVE Friends and Family 38

           Aunt Carol Rubin 40
           Psychiatrist William Packard 43
           Rabbi Gerald I. Wolpe 44
           Two Brothers—Different Perspectives
               Robert Solomon 45
               Michael Solomon 48
           Judy Solomon—A Wife's Viewpoint 50

THIRTEEN Helping Yourself and Others 55

FOREWORD
By Gloria Hochman

I met Michael Solomon 30 years ago when I was reporting on what was then called manic-depressive illness for *The Philadelphia Inquirer*. At the time, his mood swings were seesawing from the heights to the depths, bounding from reckless ecstasy to morbid despair. But his charm and personality, like many people with his condition, made his friends and family describe him this way:

- a special and delightful nephew
- a warm and caring friend
- an extraordinarily admirable human being

Several years ago, after I had co-authored with the late actor Patty Duke, the New York Times bestselling book, "*A Brilliant Madness,* Michael contacted me. He had come full circle, he told me, and was now working as a certified peer specialistt for people dealing with mental illness. He had struggled to turn his life around and had become a sought-after leader in the self-help movement which he is convinced can be instrumental in moving people like him toward recovery.

I was not surprised. I knew that those with mood disorders often have the capacity to tap into a rich and mysterious resource deep inside themselves, one that gives them a unique ability to translate the world in new ways and be persistent in the face of hardship and rejection.

Studies have shown repeatedly that creative people tend to have a mix of characteristics—intelligence, independence and sensitivity, combined with empathy for others and a personality style that allows them to be more adventurous and willing to take risks.
So many gifted and talented people—actor Patty Duke, composer Robert Schumann, theatrical director and producer Joshua Logan; statesman Winston Churchill; artist Vincent Van Gogh--suffered from bipolar illness.

Michael demonstrates his own brand of giftedness, generated by his intensity and his sensitivity for others. He has become a luminary in the self-help movement; he is determined to spread the word that, along with appropriate medication and psychotherapy, working in a group with a charismatic leader, can be powerful and effective. He is sharing his story so others like him will begin their journey toward mental health and fulfillment of their dreams.

MY FRIEND, MICHAEL

By Richard C. Baron. M.A.

I met Mike at a Pennsylvania Mental Health Conference several years ago. The after-dinner speaker had called in sick, and a small group of those attending had pulled together an impromptu talent show.

One person managed to recall from his high school years a ten-minute dramatic presentation from *Flowers for Algernon.* Someone else sang *Fire and Rain,* which had become the mental health movement's theme song. I seem to remember someone else with a guitar and a round of off-color lyrics. But I thought the best performance was Mike's, doing an imaginary blind date phone call, he said, in a world in which the usual prejudices about mental illness didn't exist

Hi, Joannie? Our mutual friend Carl suggested I give you a call and see if you'd be interested in going out with me one night next week.

What am I like? Well, I'm pretty tall, with brown hair that's usually unruly, and I'm still a smoker. I like sports—always wanted to be a sportscaster—and I sell life insurance and I like good food and funny movies. I'm manic-depressive, a good dancer, and I'm a pretty good friend.

Well, why don't we meet for coffee then? Tomorrow at 7? Great!

I thought that was hilarious and honest: the endless search for just the right woman in his life (someone finally showed up), the casual mention of manic-depression as just one of several characteristics—but not the most important one, and not the deal breaker.

Mike and I have been friends ever since, and he is in fact a very good friend—to me, to his family, and to his colleagues in the mental health consumer movement, and—well, actually and a little annoyingly—to every waiter and waitress in every restaurant, pizza joint and hot dog stand we've been to over the years. He's interested in people and he goes beyond his own struggles to connect to them. I think he'll connect to you, too, as you read his story.

Hello...I'm Michael Solomon

I'm 62 and I've been in a psychiatric hospital 25 times. Some of those in-patient stays came even before I was diagnosed with what was then called manic-depression.

Through my twenties and thirties, I grappled with unpredictable bouts of mania and depression and their impact on my relationships, my independence and my career.

I consider it almost a miracle that for more than 20 years I've been living a normal, healthy life, aware every day of what I need to do to maintain my mental health. I've been happily married since June 3, 2007. My mission during this time has been and continues to be as a beacon for the nearly 7 million people in this country who struggle with what is known today as bipolar illness.

Take this journey with me, and I promise that you will learn as I have how to live with hope and move toward the productive life you may believe is out of your reach.

Chapter One
What Is Bipolar Illness Anyway?

I know that everyone has times when they feel "blue," when they want to pull the covers over their heads and shut out the world…other times when they feel as though they could conquer the world. This is normal. What I lived through for more than 43 years is not. It is no wonder that I couldn't get a handle on what was wrong with me. I've learned that there are so many varieties of bipolar illness that, depending on what part of your manic-depressive cycle you are in when the doctor sees you, he or she might not recognize your condition, at least not at first.

Bipolar illness is a devastating mood disorder that can take a toll on your ability to function, to hold a job, to be in a successful relationship. It is different from unipolar depression, which affects as many as 15 million men, women and even children, and feels like a black cloud which will never turn into daylight.

The National Institute of Mental Health defines bipolar illness as "episodic." Those with the condition swing from mania to depression with periods of normalcy in-between.

In the depressive state, you may feel sad, anxious and hopeless. You're slowed down, have trouble concentrating, experience little energy, have trouble sleeping or need to sleep all the time. I know. I've had all those symptoms.

I can tell you about mania, too. That feels great, as though there is nothing you can't do. You talk fast, your words often tripping over each other as you try to articulate them. You have poor judgment, insatiable sexual drive, racing thoughts and find you can function on little sleep. You also deny that anything is wrong.

Not everyone with bipolar illness experiences all of the symptoms. Not everyone buys an airplane, as Patty Duke did, and leaves it running at the gate. Nor does everyone who feels depressed become suicidal. I'm going to tell you what it has been like for me, how it feels to live with a mental illness.

Mental health experts say it is not, as is often believed, something a person can control on his own. It is primarily a medical condition that results from abnormal brain chemistry—an imbalance of brain chemicals called neurotransmitters. Some of these chemicals related to mood disorder are serotonin, dopamine and norepinephrine. That's why I call my book "It Comes From Within." Fortunately, because it is a brain disorder, it is usually treatable although there may likely be a period of trial and error with a variety of medications. Unfortunately, just a little more than a quarter of those afflicted never get professional help. I hope this book will change that.

Chapter Two
How Did I Get This Way?

Some people insist that bipolar illness has its genesis in a chaotic, dysfunctional early childhood. This is not my experience. I was lucky to have grown up in a comfortable, loving family—my father, Abraham Martin Solomon, over six feet tall with a receding hairline and generous with his hugs; my mom, Sylvia Dorothy Rubin (her maiden name), one of five children, my older siblings—my brother Robert and my sister Carol. By the time I was born, my father had a more flexible schedule from his job as a food broker...and more time to spend with me, his "magic baby." One of my most vivid memories is that of me always making his breakfast even if it was just cereal and milk. The nourishment we gave each other was more love than food. My dad was my God. If I made him happy, I was happy.

As soon as I learned to read, I began studying the sports section of the newspapers. I couldn't wait until Sundays when my dad, who had season tickets, and I drove to Franklin Field for the Eagles football games. We were frequent visitors, too, to Connie Mack Stadium where the Phillies swung the bat. I saw Sandy Koufax in a no hitter. I loved basketball and hockey too, and met Billy Cunningham, the only person in the 76ers history to win a championship first as a player, then as a coach. I envisioned that someday I would become a sportscaster.

As I grew up, my life was good, filled with love, sports and the synagogue. My father was president of B'nai Jeshurun in our Philadelphia neighborhood. He was what in Yiddish is known as a "macher," which means that he made things happen. I had been playing basketball in the neighborhood since I was a little kid...and I was good at it. So my dad found a way to set up a basketball court in the synagogue—two portable baskets in a room with lots of space and a good floor. He was the champion for the formation of a synagogue league in which I became a stickout player by the time I was 11 or 12. Our league won two championships in a row. Basketball was a highlight for me. I could have starred in the movie, "White Men Can't

Jump." My dad always said that I was the Jewish hope to become the next Wilt Chamberlain.

Ironically, although my family was devoted to Judaism, we grew up eating pork and bacon because that was my father's business. He once took a picture of my brother in the kitchen with a can of ham in the background. By accident it showed up in his Bar Mitzvah album.

Nonetheless, when I was 13, I became a Bar Mitzvah, in the traditional Jewish ceremony signifying that a boy has now become a man, that he can be part of a minyan in the synagogue. My family beamed as I recited the prayers. I had been given the choice of a big Bar Mitzvah party or a family trip to Los Angeles. I chose the trip, which we took three years later. But we still had a Sunday party. Because I was sick for the week before my Bar Mitzvah, my dad brought a barber in to cut my hair. And before the party, he filled the refrigerator with cans of imported ham, just to be funny.

When I was two, my father became an independent food broker selling pork and turkey, an occupation that continued until his death. I began working with him, and he sent me on my first plane trip to visit two manufacturers in Iowa.

I loved my immediate and my extended family. My Uncle Max was an honest Republican politician who never imposed his views on the family. It was partly because of him that I became a people person who loved public speaking. Uncle Max was a delegate for Ronald Reagan when he was running for President, he was president of Old York Road Temple in Abington, a Philadelphia suburb and was commissioner, treasurer and a tax collector of Abington Township. And he had a good heart. I've heard that if someone couldn't afford to pay his taxes, Uncle Max would pay them for him. I was so proud to be his nephew.

But it wasn't only Uncle Max who made me feel good about myself. Because of my outgoing personality, I was the favorite nephew to all of my uncles. Uncle Al took me to play golf. Uncle Norm was my buddy and always there for me. "Come on over," he would urge me. "We'll watch the Eagles together."

If my outgoing personality and love for people have its origin in my extraordinary family, it was Kate Jackson, our family housekeeper, who instilled in me my disdain for prejudice and support for people of color. Kate was like a surrogate mother to me.

This was a time of racial turmoil in our country and I was deeply affected by it even though I wasn't mature enough to understand what was happening in the world. Dr. Martin Luther King was assassinated in Memphis, Tennessee. Our middle class neighborhood was turned upside down when a radical African-American family who owned and used guns moved in. I was slapped in the schoolyard by two black teenagers who stole a small amount of money from my pocket.

I remember hugging Kate and feeling soothed as I watched her meticulously iron my shirts and pants.

Later in life, Kate became a caregiver for her son Noel who was paralyzed in the Korean War. I visited him with her at the Veterans' Hospital in West Philadelphia. Kate introduced me to the staff as "my Michael."

Against my background of love and nurturing, it was no wonder that I did well in school and made friends easily, I even became first lieutenant of the school's safety patrol. I lived what you might call a blissful life. Until I was 14.

I know now that depression and bipolar illness often run in families, that its mystery is encoded in the genes. That's why doctors who treat this condition take a thorough family history. In my case, the genetic markers are subtle, but significant. My grandmother May and my grandfather Barney, on my father's side, were first cousins. They had four sons, none of whom exhibited symptoms. But on my mother's side of the family, her first cousin's son, Sandor, is living with schizophrenia.

Environment contributes too. My mom's family—the Rubins--- suffered a devastating loss, which shaped their dynamics. Uncle Phillip, my mom's oldest brother, a promising athlete, was hit in the head by a baseball and died when he was 16. Uncle Eddie, my mom's twin brother, lived with a high-functioning form of mental retardation. How much all of this has to do with my mental illness is something no one can know with certainty.

But I know that life changed for me when our family moved to a tony suburb just outside Philadelphia, where I became a ninth grade student in a new middle school. The other kids, most of whom had known each other for years, shunned me. They called me "Stinky Solomon." It wasn't until I learned that I had bad breath caused by instant breakfast with coffee-flavored milk that I knew what precipitated the name-calling. I was too ashamed to tell my parents, so I just repressed my emotions.

But basketball became my ticket to respect. I made the varsity team as a ninth grade newcomer. And yet, I yearned for my old neighborhood, Mount Airy, and my father would drive me there frequently to play football with my old buddies.

In the fall of 1970, when I was 15 and playing tackle football without pads, my left knee was crushed by an illegal block from behind. I spent a week in the hospital enduring excruciating pain followed by most of tenth grade on crutches. I didn't know then that this physical pain would pale compared to the emotional turmoil that lie ahead, with behavior I couldn't control and an illness that doctors couldn't seem to eradicate.

Chapter Three
Looking Backward

I couldn't re-join the Harriton Rams Varsity Basketball team because my leg wasn't fully healed. Instead, I turned my attention to having fun. I spent weekends with my brother at George Washington University, visited my cousin Mitchell and had a chain of blind dates with my cousin Jodee's high school friends. I passed my driving test which made me feel grown up and in charge of myself and the world. Like many of my contemporaries, I learned how to cut classes without getting caught. You might say I was a rule breaker.

I skipped my senior prom which happened to fall on a Friday, opting instead for my standing pinochle date with Pop-Pop Barney, my fathers and uncles Mark, Mike and Willey. On Saturdays, Uncle Mike, my dad and I played indoor tennis.

Then came a crisis. My parents found a small amount of pot in my room. It had been gifted to me by a friend to thank me for a ride home. It was the first time I had it…and wouldn't you know, they found it. They were stunned and kept changing their minds about whether I could be trusted to leave home for Boston University, the college of my choice. Finally, with urging from my brother-in-law, they allowed me to go.

School was stressful because I wasn't academically prepared. Partying and intramural sports were more of a priority than scholastics during my freshman year. Somehow I managed to eek out a 2.58 average my first semester. But when I came home for Thanksgiving, I learned that a close friend and neighbor had burned to death in an explosion at work. So, instead of a turkey and pumpkin pie dinner with my family we all went to a funeral and a Shiva (the Jewish mourning period observed after a death).

My First Depression

When I flew back to school, I couldn't stop thinking about my friend and the tragic way he died. I wrote a paper about it, about the Shiva and the effect it was having on me. My social sciences professor said it was too emotional for him to even give me a grade, and suggested I present it to my friend's family. Meanwhile, I was broadcasting sports features on the school's radio station. But it didn't keep me from obsessing about my friend's untimely and painful death.

Then, it all began to fall apart. I lost it. I was pulling all-nighters, playing board games and wandering around campus in the darkness of night. I was beyond despondent, and finally left Boston to come home.

But being home didn't even begin to chip away at my depression. I couldn't get out of bed in the morning because I couldn't face the day. I felt as though I were carrying a heavy weight on my shoulder. If someone had given me a choice between depression and heart surgery, I'd have taken heart surgery in a minute.

Then something new…and frightening…happened. My thoughts kept racing beyond my control and I couldn't hold a conversation. My words made no sense and they tumbled over each other in a way that no one could understand. My high school friends abandoned me because I was acting so crazy. And my parents were mystified…they didn't know what was going on.

They rushed me to Dr. Larry Kravitz, the first in what would become a chain of psychiatrists that would form the network of my life. I remember sitting in his office, struggling to tell him what I was feeling. Instead, I put my head on his desk and cried like a baby.

****

Michael didn't know yet that he would be diagnosed with bipolar disorder. It is a condition often difficult to identify because there is no definitive laboratory test, no x-ray that can confirm this illness. It is like trying to diagnose a heart attack without an electrocardiogram.

Bipolar illness, too, comes in many forms. Not everyone experiences it the way Michael did. At one time, when it was typically called manic-depressive illness, it was thought to be a condition only of psychotic highs and suicidal lows that could swing its victims between feeling they could conquer the world and convincing them that life is not worth living. It does not always follow a predictable course. Some people mainly feel depressed with just a few manic episodes. Others have just the opposite—mainly manias punctuated with a sprinkling of depressive periods.

Then there is the mystifying "dysphoric mania" — hyperactivity and colliding ideas laced with irritability and apathy. In Europe and increasingly in this country, even recurrent cycles of depression are often thought to be a form of bipolar illness.

The classic form, though not the most prevalent, is called by the medical professions "bipolar I." When they are manic, people with this form of the illness may do outrageous, outlandish things. They may plan a yearlong trip around the world even though their bank account registers empty; buy three new cars even though they don't drive, agree to marry today someone they met at last night's party. They feel invincible and see no consequences for their behavior. They have relentless energy and can survive on amazingly little sleep. A 54-old woman remembers that she would have dozens of ideas and feel she could implement them all the next day--paint her entire apartment, write a script for a new television sitcom, invite everyone on her floor for dinner even though she didn't cook and couldn't afford to order in. "I thought my ideas were brilliant...and doable," she says.

In extreme mania, people's judgment vanishes, they spend money extravagantly (the late actor Patty Duke bought a dune buggy although she didn't drive and had no use for it). They make ill-conceived business deals, may gamble away their daughter's college education fund and become outraged quickly. They become hypersexual, and tangled words and sentences that make no sense spill out of their mouths. No wonder they wear out their family and friends.

People who are going through the depressive cycle of bipolar illness feel the same gloom as those who are experiencing major depression. They can't make decisions, have difficulty concentrating, lose interest in sex and feel hopeless, as though life will never be bright again. One woman said, "All of you is in pain. Even your hair hurts."

No one knows how many people suffer from bipolar II. Here there are no sharp highs and lows, just recurring depressions without psychotic manic episodes. Instead, they may experience "hypomanic" periods, during which they may be astonishingly productive. A car salesman will sell more cars. An artist will paint more paintings (Vincent van Gogh with his startling bursts of energy punctuated by tragic depressions was thought by many to have suffered from bipolar II); an author may complete a book in three days.

"Their minds work faster, they may be sharper, even sharper-tongued," says Dr. Hagop Akiskal, a specialist in the disorder. "Even though they take risks and sometimes act impulsively, they are charming and intense and generate a sense of excitement." Unfortunately, there is a price to pay. These productive episodes often come at the end of a debilitating depression during which time they have accomplished nothing.

Bipolar II's are brutal to live with. Their excessive exuberance can be wearing and their shifts into gloom jolting.

Chapter Four
A Rocky Road Ahead

Dr. Kravitz thought I was suffering from depression and prescribed a medication called Stelazine which was supposed to glue my head together. That might have worked if I were a model airplane. But for me, it seemed to have the opposite effect. In fact, my sadness became so deep that I overdosed on this drug to escape from life. But it wasn't a real suicide attempt because I knew my beloved mother was in the next room and would not let me die. She and my dad raced me to nearby Lankenau Hospital where I had my first psychiatric admission.

Although it was clear I couldn't return to school in Boston where I would be living on my own, I was glued together enough to enroll in Temple University in downtown Philadelphia to study radio, TV and film. It didn't last long. I felt like a lost soul; during my two semesters there, I wasn't getting much sleep, and before long, manic symptoms began to surface. I did one brief sports report on the school's radio station, but I was in bad shape and couldn't keep it up. In retrospect, I was probably cycling, but at the time I didn't even know what the word meant.

My next stop was American University in Washington DC where I lived in a friend's dingy basement apartment and commuted to school. My friend's father had died recently, but I was more depressed than he was. Nonetheless, I enrolled in a journalism course and was accepted to do play-by-play for the university's basketball games. Jim Lynam was then head coach. His career later took him to Philadelphia where he became coach, then general manager of the Philadelphia 76ers.

I should have been happy. But it wasn't up to me. Something inside me that I couldn't identify or control was robbing me of my ability to think clearly and make sound decisions. My depressive and manic periods became so debilitating that I dropped out of this school too. I tried to drive home from Washington without a penny in my pocket. Since I had no money for tolls, my father got a phone call at each stop to verify that he would be responsible for the charges. By the time I got home, I felt like a lost soul, and my parents knew I was mentally ill.

Somehow, they got me to the Carrier Clinic, a behavioral healthcare system in Belle Mead, New Jersey that specialized in psychiatric treatment. I spent 30 days there without visitors, which was hard on me and my mom because I was her "magic baby."

But my time there turned out to be kind of fun. We had group meetings and individual therapy. There was a coffee shop where we could get burgers and milk shakes. I was observed daily and was under the care of an extraordinary psychiatrist, Ervin Varga.

One day, he sat me down, looked straight into my eyes and said the words that gave me hope. "You have an illness, and it's called manic depression. There is medication that can help you feel better." I could have jumped out of my chair and hugged him. I was so happy that there was a name for what I had, and, even more, that it was treatable. That was in 1975. He prescribed lithium, a medication often effective with people who had what I had.

For one year, I felt normal…and wonderful. No crazy highs. No days pulling the cover up over my head. Then, out of nowhere, it seemed, something inside me changed the rules.

I was working at my dad's food brokerage company, and talked on the telephone frequently with a female business associate in North Carolina who sounded especially sensual to me. An insistent voice in my head— and remember that those of us who are bipolar are hypersexual—told me I had to leave immediately (it was 2 in the morning) to meet the woman behind the voice. I drove as far as Washington D.C where my brother lived, and realized that I was falling asleep at the wheel. My dad's business partner drove down to rescue me and see to it that I got home safely. Later in life, I did meet her in Siler City, North Carolina the home of another pork packer with which my father had connected.

Chapter Five
My Worst Manic Episode

I can only describe it like driving a car without brakes.

I took off on a shopping spree to Atlantic City, checking into the glitzy Resorts International Hotel, gambling, tipping big and romping wildly on the beach. I was convinced that I was the Messiah and that television stations were there to record my extraordinary adventures. My thoughts were totally scattered, and I made a lot of long distance telephone calls. By the grace of God, one of them went to my Aunt Carol and Uncle Norm Rubin.

Uncle Norm was my emergency brake. Without missing a beat, he drove from his home in Media, PA to Atlantic City at 3 in the morning to take me to his house and recover from this terrifying episode.

For most of the next four years I was an on again, off again patient at the Philadelphia Psychiatric Center, now Belmont Hospital.

After that, a regular regimen of lithium— over 2000 mg a day—kept me somewhat stable. In 1977, the manager of radio station WNAR whom I had met at my grandfather's (PopPop Rubin) Shiva, gave me a volunteer job doing high school football reports. I even became the color analyst for the Radnor-Lower Merion game, one of the oldest high school rivalries in the country. Meanwhile, I received a diploma in liberal arts from Villanova University, while I worked as an intern producer on CBS sports radio. My dad gave me a job in his business, and I moved to my own apartment.

In 1980, as part of my studies and worth six credits, I spent a summer in Spain, outlasting my fellow students at a bloody bullfight and speaking Spanish with ease to the fans. I thought I was doing pretty well, and said to myself, as many people like me do, "You don't need lithium anymore."

So I just stopped taking it. And, of course, I began to unravel. The first thing that went was my sense of judgment. I became angry for reasons I couldn't explain, and would go from feeling normal one minute to smashing my patio table the next. I wasn't sleeping at night. I started chasing women—a gorgeous waitress for whom I wrote a poem; an adorable little Italian girl who lived in Prospect Park. I'd wake up an hour-and-a-half early just to take her to her class at court reporting school.

Next came Vicky who worked at a dress shop and had an incredible figure. With her, I had my first sexual encounter.

But it was Janis, whom I met through my brother-in-law, who taught me everything I never knew about sex. At first it was lust, not love, that defined our relationship. But I loved her family, and eventually I thought I loved her too. In 1982, I bought her an engagement ring. My mother tried to dissuade her from marrying me because of the unsettling nature of my illness. Janis knew about my condition, but I guess her love was blind. A year later, on June 25, 1983 we got married **at** the Oxford Circle Jewish Community Center in northeast Philadelphia.

It was a huge wedding—250 people. I had the most heated argument with my father about the number of guests. He wanted to invite 100 more people. The wedding was beautiful, and I was so happy. I thought my life was settled. I had a wife, a job and I felt normal. Unfortunately, it didn't last long.

Chapter Six
My Dad Can't Die, Can He?

Near the end of 1985, my world crumbled. My dad, my best friend, my boss and my role model…was diagnosed with cancer and was given nine months to live. I was devastated and angry, and I totally unraveled. First, I left my wife. For no good reason. Then I quit Dad's business because of multiple disagreements with the long-time office manager. Luckily for me, a friend, my guardian angel, Robert Montgomery, came to my temporary rescue. He gave me a job in his gas and service station and lent me the money for a "Get," a religious divorce in the Jewish tradition. I don't think to this day that Janis realizes that my leaving her was not her fault. So many irresponsible decisions!

I was scared, and somehow I felt that a spirit world was trying to speak to me. It was a terrible time for me-with my dad sick, with Janis gone, without the structure of my work in our family business.

I can't even recall the specific incident that brought it on, but I wound up at Haverford State Hospital for 30 days. I had a great social worker there, and we focused on my reaction to my dad's illness. I kept having mood swings while trying to think about my dad's philosophy that "everything works out for the best." There was no way I could accept that. I didn't see anything good in my future. I wanted to get out of Haverford and that's as far as my vision could go.

My head was in a bad place, but the focus of my family was on dad, not on me. It was only with the help of two friends that I was able to leave Haverford and move to New Foundations, a halfway house in Bryn Mawr, Pennsylvania.

While I was living there, on July 25, 1986, my father died. It came as no surprise that it was a major setback for me. My brother handled all the details of the funeral, which was overflowing with people because my dad was so well known in the food industry. As you can imagine, I was in bad shape. I remember that it was hot at his funeral, that my cousin Ross kept bringing me water, which I needed because the lithium I was taking made me incredibly thirsty. I couldn't stop sobbing.

It was the perfect time –wouldn't you know it--to make another in my chain of bad decisions. I decided to leave New Foundations and move into my own apartment in Norristown, closer to a self-help program I had been asked to lead by the Behavioral Health Administrator for Montgomery County. The program was called S.H.A.R.E. (Self Help, Advocacy and Resource Exchange). The thought was that those with bipolar illness could benefit from a facilitator who had experienced the condition.

The job didn't work out. I can't remember whether I was fired or quit, but I was so frustrated and stressed, and probably cycling between mania and depression, that I set a fire in a trash can outside the S.H.A.R.E. office in Bridgeport, Pennsylvania. I didn't mean it to spread inside the building, but it did, and the police were called.

Chapter Seven
Life in Psychiatric Centers

I was committed to Norristown State Hospital where I spent three-and-a-half months. My Uncle Norm was my sole visitor, and he came only once. I remember that he brought me pizza and gave me some money. This was the darkest time in my life. My psychiatrist, Robert Miller who looked like Kojac on TV, was my only beacon of hope. He knew how sick I was, but he respected my intelligence. He never gave up on me.

For the next five years, I continued to ricochet from giddy highs to wretched despair. Still on lithium, I was an in-and-out patient at Bryn Mawr and Belmont Hospitals. At my wit's end, I insisted on shock treatments. Anything that would keep me stable. I try not to think about them now, but I remember that they were terrifying. You lie on this gurney and small pads are placed on your head. You go under quickly, they zap you and you wake up with a pounding headache. They told me that small electrical currents had passed through my brain, which had triggered a brief seizure. The procedure would hopefully cause changes in my brain chemistry that would relieve my symptoms. I had four treatments. A far as I could tell, they didn't hurt, but they didn't help either.

My next stop in 1991 was the psychiatric unit at the Hospital of the University of Pennsylvania. Doctors there took me off lithium because of potential side effects such as kidney damage. They replaced it with yet another medication, something called Depakote.

My mother had been a widow for six years by now, still struggling with how to live without my father. She barely recognized who I had become, shuttling a couple of times a year in and out of psychiatric facilities. I desperately wanted to ease the pain for both of us and finally end those yearly psychiatric admissions.

It was my time at the Horsham Clinic, a private in-patient hospital in Ambler, Pennsylvania, that began to turn my life around. Psychiatrist

Carl Hammer, whom a social worker at the Clinic had urged me to see, prescribed a new medication, Clozaril.

Thankfully, Clozaril seemed to even me out, and my emotional healing began.

Chapter Eight
Treatments that Transform

If you've ever enjoyed a mineral water bath such as those in posh resorts like Saratoga, New York or Calistoga, California, you probably remember how thoroughly relaxed you felt for hours afterward. That's because you were bathing in water that contains lithium, a healing substance. Patients with what used to be called "nervous breakdowns" have often been sent to bathe in mineral baths to soothe their anxieties.

Today, lithium is considered a wonder drug for those with bipolar illness. It has the power to restore normalcy to 60 to 70 percent of those for whom it is prescribed. It was used in other countries in the early fifties, but was not recognized in America until more than a decade later.

Dr. Ronald Fieve, a New York psychiatrist, was a pioneer in championing the use of lithium for those with bipolar illness. In 1958, he conducted clinical research trials of lithium in the acute ward of the New York Psychiatric Institute and became convinced that lithium was an almost magical treatment for those with the condition. After it was studied by doctors in Texas who agreed with Dr. Fieve, the results were presented to those attending the annual meeting of the American Psychiatric Association in May, 1965. It took another six years for lithium to receive a FDA endorsement as a maintenance medication for bipolar illness.

The appropriate lithium dose is often trial and error until the effective therapeutic level is reached. Twenty percent of those who take it regularly are relieved of all symptoms. Another 50 percent improves substantially. Michael was not one of the lucky ones. He was one of the 30 percent who couldn't be sustained on lithium although initially it seemed to modify his highs and lows.

For Michael and others like him, another medication added to the lithium often achieves what lithium itself cannot do. When that doesn't work, a potpourri of other medications and treatments can be effective.

An anticonvulsive drug—Tegretol—used originally to control seizures or epilepsy because it settles abnormal impulses in the brain, is especially helpful for those who have acute mania or the overlapping symptoms of both mania and depression.

Other drugs in this category include valproate (Depakote, Depakene) or Clonazepam (Klonopin) which is usually prescribed in small doses because of its sedating effect. Clozapine (Clozaril) is an anti-psychotic medication that may be given for the psychotic symptoms of mania, but those taking it are, after about three weeks, usually able to wean off the drug and transition to lithium alone.

In extreme cases, different types of treatment technologies frequently help. Electroconvulsive therapy (ECT), for example, was not effective for Michael but for many patients, it is almost magical. It is usually done as an inpatient or day hospital procedure. It is always administered with anesthesia and muscle relaxants, and is generally given two or three times a week over a several-week period. Controlled and carefully calculated doses of electrical currents are delivered to the brain while heart rate and blood pressure are monitored. ECT is considered to be the most effective treatment for severe depression that has been unresponsive to other modalities. The most common side effects are confusion and memory loss.

The US Food and Drug Administration, in March, 2018, approved Lurasidone for the treatment of major depressive episodes associated with bipolar I in children and adolescents ages 10 to 17. It was already approved to treat adults with bipolar depression.

A Little Humor

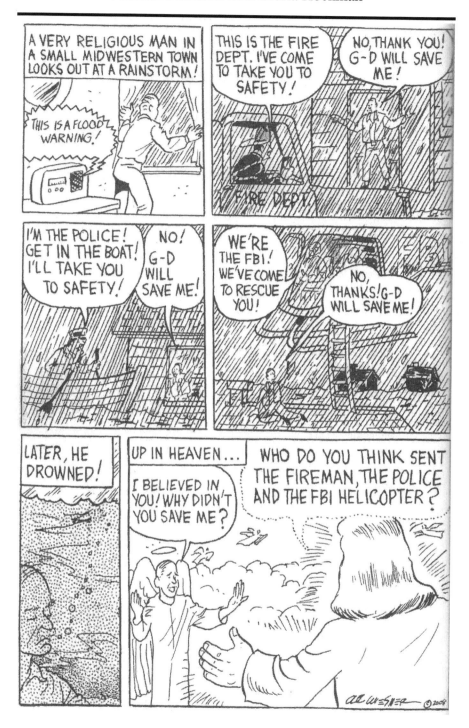

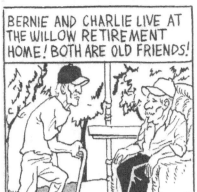

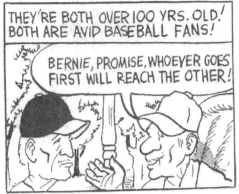

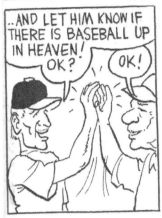

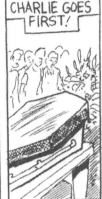

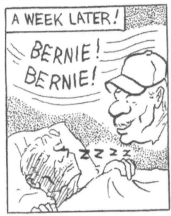

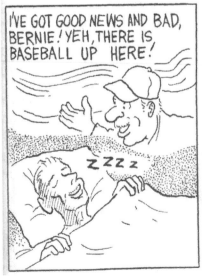

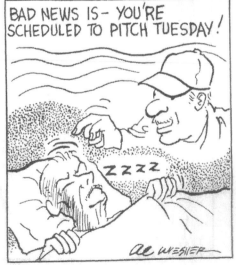

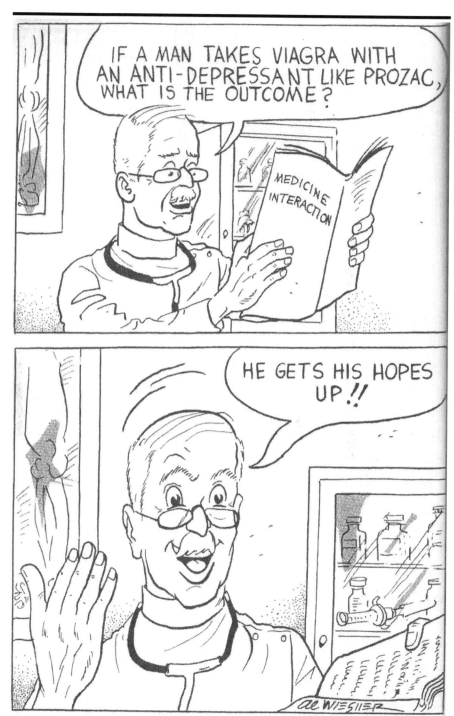

Chapter Nine
A New Start

My mom bought me a one-bedroom condominium, at auction, in a quiet western suburb, and I was enjoying having my own place and taking care of it.

I wanted to return to Judaism which had once been a significant segment of my life, and I wanted to be part of a community of worshipers. I checked out orthodoxy, but it wasn't for me. So I walked across the street to Har Zion synagogue, not realizing that first step would change my life.

I started reading the Old Testament, and realized that until I was 31, my father had been my God. Now it was time to seek the real God. I was returning to my religion, Judaism, and my faith in God was reborn. I remembered that God spoke to Moses, and I think that God speaks to us through the people we meet.

I was lucky enough to meet Judy when we were both members of our amateur synagogue choir. Judy has a beautiful voice, mine not so much. Judy had just ended a long-term relationship, and our friendship developed slowly. We both participated in two plays at our synagogue, and enjoyed each other's company.

But life, of course, doesn't go smoothly…and stress is unavoidable. In 2002, in spite of my growing relationship with Judy, another woman was calling me constantly and showing up unexpectedly at my door. Meanwhile, Judy was pressuring me to get ready for her nephew's wedding—she gave me a week.

The combined stress resulted in my return to poor judgment. This is what happened. Shortly after midnight on March 22, 2002, I managed to set my apartment on fire. I had been testing the smoke alarm, and it ignited.

The police were called, and an officer whisked me, in handcuffs, to Montgomery County Emergency Services where I was considered to be in an acute manic state. It was noted that I had been hospitalized for mental illness in Bryn Mawr Hospital seven years earlier and had a medical record crammed with inpatient admissions. At a hearing five days later, I remember saying, "I'm human. I'm allowed to make a mistake." Nonetheless, I was turned over without my consent, to Bryn Mawr Hospital's psychiatric unit where I was diagnosed with psychosis and paranoia.

I didn't want my mother to know what happened because I knew how much it would upset her. So I told her I was taking a brief vacation. To be sure I wouldn't be found out, I called my friend Warren Levy, another of my guardian angels. Warren lived in the same condominium I did and had a key to my apartment. I instructed him to go in and disconnect my telephone answering machine, which is something I would have done if I were indeed going on vacation. Even though I was grappling with mental demons, I was lucid enough to want to protect my family.

My psychiatrist, William Packard, who was on vacation at the time, didn't think I had received the correct diagnosis. He called what I had done an acute and temporary manic episode, one from which I would recover quickly. He was right; I left Bryn Mawr in eight days.

Still, I continued my personal game of keeping all of this a secret from my friends and family. When I was released, it was Warren who picked me up and my "vacation" was almost over.

A year later, my mother was diagnosed with cancer, a condition with which she wrestled for the next several years. Nonetheless, for my 50th birthday, she insisted on treating me to a trip to Israel. At the Wailing Wall, I posted a note asking the Lord to be gentle with my mother's soul.

When I returned home, I learned that my mother's cancer which had seemed to be under control, had resurfaced and was inoperable. Her loss, four weeks later, was jolting and devastating. But she died

31

peacefully without pain killers, surrounded by her loved ones. That indicated to me that my note on the Wailing Wall had not gone unheeded. I believed that our Creator was indeed gentle with my beloved mother's soul.

I took time to compose myself before mom's funeral. At the service, I couldn't say all that I wanted to. In the midst of tears streaming down my cheeks, I told those who had come to pay their respect, "In love, mom and dad created Carol, Robert and me…and their love will endure forever."

Judy and I got married June 3, 2007. As you will read in Judy's message, it hasn't always been easy. But we have a strong emotional and spiritual connection. Judy is not only my wife, but also my best friend. Any sexual activity is like the icing on a cake or mushrooms on a pizza.

Chapter Ten
The Power of Peers...the Miracle of Friendship

I'm resigned to being dependent on medication to maintain my stability and judgment—2 mg of Klonopin and 200 mg of Clozaril every day. I'm resigned to taking blood tests every month to check any side effects from the medications. I know that I'll have trouble sleeping at night if I don't swallow them before bedtime, and, believe me, you don't want to be with me if I'm sleep-deprived.

I know that stress is the big trigger for me. So is a lost night's sleep. Skipping a meal. These are my self-imposed rules:

- Drive without the distraction of a radio so I can stay focused
- Get 10 hours of sound sleep a night
- Work diligently at maintaining my happy marriage
- Rely on support from my faith-based community
- Reduce the number of my daily activities to avoid stress, and carve out ample time to accomplish each.
- Keep my finances as simple as possible.

But I also know that becoming involved in the mental health consumer movement—first as a mental health patient, then as an educator, a speaker, an organizer and leader of self-help groups—has done as much or more to rescue me from the vicious cycle of bipolar illness.

As far back as 1986, a friend of my mother's had connected me with someone who was facilitating a self-help support group for the Mental Health Association of Southeastern Pennsylvania, now Mental Health Partners. It met every Tuesday either at the Philadelphia Medical Institute in center city or the Philadelphia Psychiatric Center (now Belmont Hospital) just out of town. The idea was that someone who had experienced the symptoms of mental illness could lead a discussion with others then going through it, being responsible for organizing the meetings, setting the agendas and presiding over them.

I was taking significant doses of lithium then, but they weren't fully controlling my manias. However, in the two years I ran the group, I learned about the power of friendship and the healing instigated by shared experiences and a strengthened ego.

Typically, someone in a support group finds comfort, strength, and hope with others like them. Family and friends can offer a shoulder to cry on and give limited encouragement, but they can't relate fully to the person who is experiencing the turmoil in their brains. An effective support group helps those in it to look beyond their own problems while making new friends and relating to people who understand. A goal is to emerge with higher self-esteem despite past failures.

I met the mom of a brilliant young man who, just after receiving a prize from his Ivy League university for best freshman achievement in mathematics, asked to come home. He was too anxious to focus on his studies. He was diagnosed first with bipolar illness, then with schizophrenia, then again with bipolar illness. After years of trying, then abandoning a medley of medications, after living in psychiatric units and halfway houses, after undergoing a series of electroshock treatments, and finally relying on his mother's unconditional support, he found his way. Today, his mom says gratefully, he is married, has two daughters and works as a substitute teacher. Participation in a self-help group keeps this mother grounded and gives hope to others.

In 1988, the Behavioral Health Administrator for Montgomery County, Pennsylvania asked me to start Project S.H.A.R.E. (Self Help, Advocacy and Resource Exchange), but before long I began to cycle again. Even my work with psychiatrist Robert Miller couldn't get me stable. Somehow-- I still don't know how—I had the mental stamina to complete a research paper I had started on, *The Success of Self-Help: Fact or Fiction.*

This research into the origin and effectiveness of self-help, coupled with my experience as both participant and leader, convinced me that this was a path to recovery for those of us with serious mental health conditions.

Chapter Eleven
Spreading the Word

In 2009, after having taken an intensive training course, I became a certified peer specialist. Today I work for Montgomery County Emergency Services. I can't tell you how empowering it feels to now have a key to the facility I used to enter only as a patient.

Today, I work for the National Alliance on Mental Illness (NAMI) in two programs. NAMI Connection focuses on peer support and recovery, and meets every other week.

And I'm the senior presenter in NAMI's crisis intervention program in Montgomery County, *"In Our Own Voice."* I present to law enforcement officers in Lower Merion and other counties, to members of FBI Homeland Security and to Human Services groups at colleges and universities. My goal is to increase awareness and understanding of mental illness and to fight stigma.

When someone asks me if people with mental illness are ever really cured, I tell them I live with a mental illness. It's a small part of my identity. To know it's only a small part is important.

I begin a new session of *"Voice"* with a DVD where the performers are not actors; they are real people living with a mental illness.

The first topic is *"Dark Days."* I tell the group about my own "dark days," when I had to leave Boston University racked with depression, overdosing on Stelazine and spending three-and-a-half months as an inpatient at Norristown State Hospital

A woman at one of my presentations revealed her own dark days. "I hid in a closet, literally," she said, "where I couldn't see or be seen, couldn't hear, or be heard, because being in the world was too scary for me."

Another woman said, "I'm a failure and a loser, an alien in this world. I feel possessed by demons Why keep trying?

"I'd rather have broken bones or deliver 15-pound twins without anesthesia than go through one bout of depression."

Claudia, a 45-year-old woman with frizzy blonde hair, confided, "I'm not in a good place right now. I need help with mental confusion caused by my serious depression. Four months ago, I was in the hospital for a suicide attempt. It helps to hear from other people who have been where I am and moved past it."

The next category is *"Acceptance."* Mine came twice. Once, just after I was diagnosed, when I realized that I had a condition that came with a name and a treatment that could probably even me out, and again in 1997 when I accepted that a lifetime commitment to medication could break my cycle of psychiatric admissions.

In the next session, *"Treatment,"* I reveal how blessed I feel to have a team in place—my psychiatrist, pharmacist, an outpatient lab for blood work, an internist, an excellent vocational counselor, and most important, a loving, stable wife.

Our fourth topic, *"Coping Skills,"* "gives me a chance to share mine: as I described earlier in this chapter-- keeping stressors to a minimum and controlling behaviors that I know will cause me trouble.

My favorite part is the one that ends the session: *"Success, Hopes and Dreams."* If you measure those goals by education, I'm proud that I have a degree from Villanova University even though it took me seven years and four colleges to get it. If you measure it by income, I know I can earn a living since I was my father's sales manager at his brokerage firm for four years.

Most important, if you define success by the number of people you've helped throughout your life, I'm a wealthy man. I've been active in the mental health field as a volunteer and paid employee for more than 30 years. Basically, I love people and I don't feel the least bit vulnerable opening up to new acquaintances, maybe because of the countless hours of hard work I've spent in therapy. Along the way, I've made cherished, invaluable friends. I like this short verse

There is a miracle called friendship that dwells within the heart

We don't know how it happens or when it gets its start.

The happiness it brings you always gives a special lift

And we realize that friendship is God's most precious gift

I especially like offering training to law enforcement officials who often come into contact with persons with severe mental illness. In fact, a report issued by the Treatment Advocacy Center and the National Sheriff's Association estimates that half the number of people shot and killed by police have mental health problems. NAMI reports that nearly two million people with mental health problems are booked into jail every year. When they encounter police, what happens to them often depends on the skills of the officers involved, their ability to recognize mental illness and deal safely and appropriately with those experiencing a psychiatric crisis.

My hope is that those who suffer from mental disorders and their families will hear me and begin to see a light, a small spark that enables them see that their lives are not hopeless, that it is possible to regain mental health and happiness.

When I talk to law enforcement officers or to anyone who does not suffer from bipolar illness, I hope they will reflect on my presentation when they encounter someone with a mental illness who is not stable. I hope they will see that troubled person as someone with the potential to live a life of recovery. My dream is for a society without stigma and any kind of prejudice, where, as my former therapist Margot Clark often said, "Normal is a word on a washing machine."

Chapter Twelve
Friends and Family

It is family and intimate friends who are most victimized by those with bipolar illness. As the cycles of mania and depression become more intense, it is they who are most affected. I remember Patty Duke telling me that she was "murder to live with." What is a husband to do when his wife takes to her bed for a month behind closed doors? Or when her mania turns to irritability and flashes of rage?

When arguments become loud and ugly and recurring, marriages often break apart. When a husband or wife is understanding and forgiving, as John Astin, Patty Duke's husband was, it often agitates the bipolar person even more.

Parents wring their hands and don't know what has come over their son or daughter. "He used to be such a special child—warm and loving and a diligent student, "says the mother of a 20-year-old who was diagnosed a year ago. "Now I don't know him. He talks constantly and makes no sense. It's like a motor running. He trashes his apartment and insults people. It's like the devil has overtaken him."

People with bipolar illness are often manipulative. They exasperate their therapists who frequently can't work with them when they are out of control.

Patty Duke's son, MacKenzie Astin, told me, "My mom can't keep a friend. She doesn't know how. You might be her best friend today. But I guarantee you that next year at this time, something will happen and you'll never hear from her again."

Patty said she empathized with family members and close friends of anyone with bipolar illness. "They are the innocent bystanders who are being ravaged by this thing. They can't begin to understand how someone can cry for three months in a row or fly off the handle at the flip of a switch. They are suffering as much as the person in depression or mania."

After diagnosis and treatment, there is a lot of healing to do. But fortunately for Michael, adherence to his medical protocol, his avoidance of known stressors and his diligent participation in self-help groups have kept him mentally healthy. He remains in a loving, if sometimes challenging, marriage and is surrounded by caring friends and family. These messages show the love that envelops him.

Aunt Carol Rubin

Michael came into my life when I started dating his Uncle Norm. I remember him as the cutest kid with curly hair, pretty blue eyes and a wide, wide smile.

The first indication that Michael was having problems came when he and his parents would come to our house for dinner. Michael was a young man then. I noticed his pale complexion and lack of expression both on his face and in his behavior. Later, the reality of Michael's burden became evident.

On a late evening in 1978, our phone rang. Our two sons, Ross who was 10 and Jon who was 7, were asleep in their rooms.

It was Michael calling from Atlantic City. I answered the phone and heard Michael telling me he was calling from one of the casinos. He asked me if I knew why he was there. I answered that I did not know. His next words sent chills down my spine. He told me he was the Messiah and the television stations were there to record this event. He told me he bought a new bicycle, and wanted his Uncle Norm to come down and meet him in the lobby of the Resorts Hotel.

Without missing a beat, Norm headed for Atlantic City and was back home two hours later with Michael who was manic and unable to sleep. He made a phone call and I heard him yelling at the person on the other end of the line; it was his father.

When the conversation was over, I went to check on Michael, and there was this huge guy who bent over to hug me. We just hugged tightly for a minute. He was no longer out of control, just overwhelmed and sad.

The next day, Norm left for a hospital with Michael in the passenger seat of his car. But the relief I felt was short-lived. Norm told me that Michael had become rather violent, banging on the dashboard yelling that he did not want to go to the hospital. Norm said he had no choice but to return home.

Later, on the recommendation of a friend, Norm took Michael to a doctor in Havertown. From there began the odyssey of many years of finding the right combination of medications that helped Michael graduate from college, become a mentor for challenged children, tutor young students for their Bar Mitzvahs. He also worked for his Uncle Norm at the Norman Rubin insurance agency.

One of the many attributes Michael has given to us is his big, generous heart. Everyone who knows Michael knows this about him. He has more friends, family and colleagues who are proud to call him a friend than anyone else I know.

Memories that "bless and burn" for Michael and our family are those where we were all watching the Eagles and agonized or cheered depending on whether they won or didn't.

Baseball, football, swimming pools, barbeques, family celebrations-- they were all the foundation of our life with our wonderful Michael Solomon. How lucky for us all that we have had Michael to teach us what it is like to come from the abyss and succeed in all he has attempted.

Michael and his wife Judy have become an integral part of the family bringing warmth, additional family to share life cycle events, and an extended sense of family.

As a matter of fact, we are reliving history. Michael is here with me watching the Eagles trying to beat the New York Giants while my vegetable soup is on the stove and the rest of the family is coming for dinner.

Life is great now that our beloved Eagles have won Superbowl 52!

William Packard, M.D.

I have been Michael Solomon's psychiatrist for 15 years. He is a man I respect and admire. He is a friend. Michael gains the respect of whatever community he serves because he is intelligent and has a big heart. He is dedicated, sincere and truly compassionate. His desire to help those who are less fortunate comes from his strong faith, which he shares with his wife. It is probably due in part to the suffering he has experienced because of his mental illness, but also the commitment that has deep roots in his family and its values.

I knew Michael from the period where he was still trying to accept his illness to the present where he teaches others to give them the insight they require to take the best care of themselves. He has suffered a great deal and it is a credit to him that he has rewritten his history.

Unfortunately, I was out of town when Michael was involuntarily committed to a psychiatric facility in 2002. He was diagnosed as being depressed. He was not. He was experiencing an acute manic episode which, like most manic episodes, is temporary. Within four days, Michael was beginning to improve; four days later he was discharged.

Michael's acute episode and his subsequent misdiagnosis, resulted in pain for him and all of those who loved him.

Michael's message to you is simple. Never feel ashamed because you have a mental illness. It is a fact of your life. Understanding it and learning from it will help you control it. Shame leads to bad decisions and unstable relationships. Knowledge is power.

The late Rabbi Gerald I. Wolpe

My awareness of those who are mentally ill and their need for understanding and support came to me because of the remarkable Michael Solomon. He comes to Har Zion services regularly, on Shabbat and holidays, and is seen at most of our educational services. Michael considers his role to be as an advocate for his own struggle against manic-depressive illness as well as for those who share his condition.

I am impressed with his passion on behalf of a group that is waging a valiant battle against their "no fault disease" while trying to become part of the synagogue and the Jewish community in general to which they can offer a great deal.

I urge anyone who can benefit from Michael's wisdom and experience to contact him. Michael is always ready to help.

Note: Rabbi Wolpe wrote these words on the front page of the Bulletin of Har Zion Temple.

Two Brothers…Different Perspectives
Robert Solomon

Michael and I were totally different from the beginning. I'm the older brother. When people ask me to describe my childhood, the answer is startlingly simple: I say I grew up afraid

I was that little kid who cried in pre-school, who was frightened by his elementary school teachers, and who was intimidated by high School academics. I had no hobbies, no passions, no redeeming qualities. I was quiet, not terribly well liked, mostly unhappy, and very scared.

Michael was the opposite. He was an appealing baby who grew to be friendly, popular and reasonably self-confident. He was a big kid who seemed to like school, and was fairly accomplished athletically. Michael, in short, was well adjusted. I was not.

His future appeared bright. Mine? Not so much.

But I had one positive trait—a will to succeed. I was scared, sure, but also stubborn and determined. I was the teenage kid who ran around our neighborhood streets in the burning heat and humidity of summer to get in shape for high school football. The neighbors who watched me trudge by would laugh and say, "What in heaven's name are you doing, Bobby?"

I was the one who doggedly pursued my studies, if not to become good at school, at least to get better (I did). I was the one who stood up to a bully in the school yard (I won). And I was the one who mustered the courage to ask a pretty girl out on a date (she said yes).

In college, I discovered an ability to learn, and ultimately graduated with honors and received a Master's Degree. I began a modestly successful career in business.

Most important, I defied my father and married a woman of my own choosing (a mistake, of course). I would make another, then finally figure this out third time around.

Michael, after showing so much promise, began showing signs of decline. His mental illness surfaced long before there were terms to define it. In the beginning, I was what you might call the supportive brother. I recall going to a Washington DC hospital emergency room more than once to either see my brother or secure his release. I listened to many late night phone calls that bordered on incoherence. I ignored the bouts of unreason.

But Michael's health, always unpredictable and erratic, continued to deteriorate, trying the patience of family and friends. Me included.

For years, we barely spoke. I had no time for my brother. I wouldn't answer his calls and our few conversations were brief and curt. It was the advent of e-mail that provided a way to re-establish contact. It was less intimate than face-to-face meetings or phone calls, but more friendly than total silence. We moved from monosyllables to sentences to paragraphs. It restored a modicum of civility to our "conversations."

Meanwhile, new drugs and treatments became available, and Michael slowly healed. He seemed to be trying harder and becoming more invested in his own care. He could still be insensitive and not trusted to keep a confidence, but he was more rational and controlled. And he seemed to be resigned to the limited nature of our interaction.

But there were two events that were life changing for Michael:
    The first was the death of our mother, Sylvia. Our mom was a tremendously concerned and supportive parent, but ever since our father's death, years earlier, she had developed with Michael what appeared to be a damaging form of co-dependency. Her death, sad as it was, seemed to liberate Michael.

The second was meeting his wife, Judy. Judy saw Michael for who he is and loved him still. Their marriage has brought structure and discipline, peace and stability to his life.

If I had my way, I would have a warmer, friendlier relationship with my brother. But accustomed as I am to family conflict, I accept what we have. I don't see a lot of growth, but at least we have contact. And who knows what the future holds?

Michael Solomon

From as far back as I can remember, I felt blessed to have Robert as a big brother. For 20 years, we were very close. We shared a room, we wrestled, we enjoyed sports and looked out for each other. I remember that my heart went out to him when his best friend betrayed him by dating his girlfriend. Instead of being compassionate, our father yelled, "Robert. Be a man!" He was a teenager at the time, a student at the prestigious Central High School in Philadelphia.

He showed remarkable discipline academically as a student and by trying out for Central's football team. I often wonder whether following Robert to high school would have helped me develop a better work ethic.

When Robert went to college at George Washington University, my monthly visits to him helped us bond even more. In 1974, just at the onset of my illness, I attended my brother's wedding despite my father's objections.

For the next 11 years, my family was forced to accept me despite my behavior because dad was domineering and I was his favorite child. In retrospect, this was dysfunctional for me because my dad's happiness was a higher priority than my own sense of well-being.

When my father was dying from cancer, my brother and uncle handled his finances, and my brother was in charge of my inheritance after dad passed away. During this time and until I became stable, my brother took more than his share of verbal abuse from me. My mania would trigger spending sprees, even on escort services, and Robert took the brunt of my outbursts especially when I needed money. I often think that if the shoe were on the other foot, how would I have reacted?

Robert did a masterful job of managing my mother's money until she died in 2006. At that time, he sent me a $5000 check for Tikvah/AJMI that was left in her will. That money has gone to create an annual award in honor of our parents. When Judy and I were married, he gave us an incredibly generous wedding gift.

I'm so proud of my big brother. He has published two books—*The Art of Client Service* and *Brain Surgery for Suits.* His honesty and integrity are unwavering.

While I've tried to make amends with Robert on numerous occasions, I imagine that the emotional wounds run too deep for a total reconciliation. We don't see much of each other in person, but I wish Robert Joel Solomon many more years of health and happiness.

Judy Solomon
A Wife's Viewpoint

If anyone had told me I'd be married to a mental patient, I'd have said they were crazy. Michael and I met in a choir at our synagogue. I love to sing and have a fairly good voice. Michael, on the other hand, joined the choir to have something different to be involved in.

I thought he was kind of cute, but I kept hanging on to a long time relationship that was going nowhere. Meanwhile, Michael's outgoing and friendly personality made him so easy to be with. He called me every day and we saw each other at services. He cared about religion and spirituality, the total opposite of the guy I had been dating. And he was fun to be around. As time went on, Michael kind of grew on me. He was the one who talked a lot and I didn't feel that I had to be "on" all the time. When my other relationship was over, Michael was there to pick up the pieces.

He proposed on December 15, 2006 and we got married six months later. But I was unprepared for a marriage with someone who had bipolar illness, and the first year was a killer. For the next 24 months, I struggled to understand someone who slept into the early afternoon, had only two small jobs and didn't seem to have much ambition. Even when I asked him to do something simple like picking up the clothes from the cleaner or emptying the trash, he didn't seem to be able to do it.

I had just retired from my teaching job of 33 years and had hoped to do something different. I was used to getting out of the house at 7 a.m. and working into the night. So Michael and I had brutal non-stop arguments. What had I gotten myself into?

I joined a NAMI "Family to Family class with other relatives of mentally ill persons. There, I learned about the effects of strong medicine and how tired it could make you. I learned that as a result of taking meds at night to promote sleep, mornings are not the ideal time to have a significant conversation. It helped.

Later I found solace in the group Tikvah/AJMI (Advocates for the Jewish Mentally Ill), where I met some amazing people. Some were relatives of mental patients; others were patients. We learned from each other.

Michael has worked hard too; he has become an entirely different person from what he was ten years ago. He works most days—speaking at colleges and hospitals, at churches and synagogues; he leads a support group at the library, and encourages the formation of chapters of the National Alliance for the Mentally Ill at colleges where there are so many students suffering from depression and bipolar illness. I'm terrified of public speaking before a crowd, but Michael thrives on it. He is an excellent speaker, knowledgeable and funny and able to interact well with his audience.

He was trained to be a leader in the field and now hopes to train others. A major project for him has been this book through which he hopes to spread the message that bipolar illness in all its forms, is treatable. He wants those who suffer from it to know that a better, more productive and satisfying life is possible for them. He is devoted to removing the stigma from mental illness.

On a personal level, he is a responsive and responsible husband. He has a great sense of humor and doesn't mind making fun of himself. I love that he is compassionate toward others, thoroughly interested in people, generous and giving.

We enjoy being together, going to the theater, to movies, out to dinner and planning how we want to spend our leisure time. We're thinking of exchanging our summer vacations at the New Jersey beach with a cruise, perhaps to Alaska. We love spending time with both of our families. As you can imagine, my family had some qualms at first— they didn't know much about bipolar illness-- but over time, their concern has developed into a love and appreciation for Michael, and we do a lot of family things together.

But spirituality is the key that binds Michael and me. I come from a religious Jewish background and love and celebrate traditions. Michael

51

is still learning the traditions and customs, but he loves to read portions from the Bible and attend services and study groups with me every Saturday. The friends we have made from our synagogue have been a source of caring and understanding.

My message to those considering life with someone who is bipolar is: Being someone's best friend as Michael and I were before we married is only the beginning. You need to learn about this illness. Read a book. Talk with the spouses or partners of those who are bipolar. Become part of a support group. Approach your relationship with a sense of humor. And be patient.

Carol Caruso
First Executive Director
NAMI of Pennsylvania, Montgomery County

I've known Michael Solomon for more than 25 years. I remember when his bipolar disorder was not controlled and he would ramble and pace endlessly. But Michael was lucky. In addition to his doctor, his mother was a powerhouse of encouragement to him and a source of constant support. Without her undying love and guidance, there may have been a different story here.

Every person's journey to recovery is different, but Michael has followed a steady path that has led to helping others. He went through extensive training as a NAMI presenter, then became an in-demand Crisis Intervention Specialist at Montgomery County Emergency Services where he has trained thousands of police, probation and correctional officers and members of Pennsylvania FBI and homeland security. As a certified peer specialist and support group leader, he courageously and entertainingly shares his story of illness and recovery. Michael demonstrates that receiving a diagnosis is not the end of the world, but the beginning of a new era of opportunities and connections.

I have worked for many years with those who struggle with mental illness and their families. I have seen the chaos and trauma those illnesses create. I have seen families torn apart and polarized because of the absence of support and education.

Mental illness, the most common of all physical ailments, is the most stigmatized. Those, like Michael, who step forward and tell their stories, are heroes as they help others accept their illnesses and move on.

We need more Michael Solomons to champion those who struggle to move on with their lives. It is a great honor knowing Michael and being a part of his network.

Unfortunately, Carol passed away on December 31, 2016. She had fought cancer with all her heart and soul, and she cried to me on the telephone just before undergoing brain surgery. I visited her at Phoenixville Hospital on her 66th birthday. She was unconscious and sleeping peacefully. Her funeral in Bridgeport, Pennsylvania was overflowing with people who came to celebrate her awesome life.
Michael Solomon

Chapter Thirteen
Helping Yourself and Others

You may not be able to help yourself until you are somewhat stabilized on medication and participating in appropriate psychotherapy. As Patty Duke said, "I don't believe anyone with manic depressive illness can truly benefit from talk therapy until the chemical balance is fixed. If that doesn't get taken care of, you can talk until you're blue in the face, you can spend billions of dollars but you'll never be helped until someone says to you, "You're manic-depressive. Take your medicine, clean up the messes you've made, and get on with your life." Before taking lithium, she said, trying to participate in therapy was "like trying to fly a jet without ever having been on a plane. There was nothing wrong with the intellectual part of my brain. I understood the words the psychiatrist was saying. They just didn't compute."

Once you are somewhat stabilized, one of the biggest stumbling blocks on the road ahead is lack of self-esteem. No wonder. After all, we have ravaged our lives and those of our loved ones. Even the most brilliant of us feel beaten down when our behavior has chipped away at so much of our promise.

To learn more about how to assess your self-esteem right now, and what you can do to feel more positive about yourself, I recommend these exercises. They helped me, and I bet they'll help you too.

HOW DO YOU FEEL ABOUT YOURSELF?

Most people feel bad about themselves from time to time. So when answering these questions, think about how you feel <u>most</u> of the time.

ASSESS YOUR OWN LEVEL OF SELF-ESTEEM	
Are you easily hurt by criticism?	☐Yes ☐No
Are you very shy or overly aggressive?	☐Yes ☐No
Do you try to hide your feelings from others?	☐Yes ☐No
Do you fear close relationships?	☐Yes ☐No
Do you try to blame your mistakes on others?	☐Yes ☐No
Do you find excuses for refusing to change?	☐Yes ☐No
Do you avoid new experiences?	☐Yes ☐No
Do you continually wish you could change your physical appearance?	☐Yes ☐No
Are you too modest about personal successes?	☐Yes ☐No
Are you glad when others fail?	☐Yes ☐No
If you answered MOST of these questions "yes", your self-esteem could probably use improvement.	

Do you accept constructive criticism?	☐Yes ☐No
Are you at ease meeting new people?	☐Yes ☐No
Are you honest and open about your feelings?	☐Yes ☐No
Do you value your closest relationships?	☐Yes ☐No
Are you able to laugh at (and learn from) your own mistakes?	☐Yes ☐No
Do you notice and accept changes in yourself as they occur?	☐Yes ☐No
Do you look for and tackle new challenges?	☐Yes ☐No
Are you confident about your physical appearance?	☐Yes ☐No
Do you give yourself credit when credit is due?	☐Yes ☐No
Are you happy for others when they succeed?	☐Yes ☐No
If you answered MOST of these questions "yes", you probably have a healthy opinion of yourself.	

Whatever the level of your self-esteem now, you can take positive steps to improve it!

HOW TO THINK POSITIVELY ABOUT YOURSELF?

Make it a point to be your own best friend. That means giving yourself?

ACCEPTANCE ✓ — Identify and accept your strengths and weaknesses – everyone has them.

HELP ✓ — Set realistic goals. Meet them by learning new skills and developing your abilities.

ENCOURAGEMENT ✓ — Take a "can-do" attitude. Set a reasonable timetable for personal goals and offer yourself encouragement along the way.

PRAISE ✓ — Take pride in your achievements, both great and small. Remember your experiences are yours alone. Enjoy them!

TIME ✓ — Take time out regularly to be alone with your thoughts and feelings. Get involved in activities you can enjoy by yourself, like crafts, reading or an individual sport. Learn to enjoy your own company.

TRUST ✓ — Pay attention to your thoughts and feelings. Act on what you think is right. Do what makes you feel happy and fulfilled.

RESPECT ✓ — Don't try to be someone else. Be proud of who you are. Explore and appreciate your own special talents.

LOVE ✓ — Learn to love the unique person you are. Accept and learn from your mistakes. Don't overact to errors. Accept your successes and failures, those who love you do.

QUESTIONS AND ANSWERS

IS IT EASY to change self-esteem?

NO. It means taking a hard look at yourself, then changing the things you don't like. This takes time, but the results will be well worth the effort. If you've tried but aren't making any progress, consider seeking help from a qualified counselor.

Does high self-esteem GUARANTEE SUCCESS?

NO, but it does guarantee feeling good about yourself and others – no matter what happens.

Can I HELP OTHERS feel better about themselves?

YES. Let your positive attitude rub off on others by offering encouragement. Help them to open up. Don't put others down. Be patient with their faults and weaknesses (everyone has them).

Does high self-esteem mean SELF-CENTEREDNESS?

NO. It's not egotism or snobbishness. These are usually false fronts for feelings of insecurity and low self-esteem. Having high self-esteem is appreciating your uniqueness so you can respond to others in positive and productive ways.

SO THINK POSITIVELY ABOUT YOURSELF

TAKE PRIDE IN YOUR INDIVIDUALITY

HELP YOURSELF BY DEVELOPING YOUR TALENTS AND ABILITIES

ENCOURAGE YOURSELF WHENEVER YOU NEED IT

PRAISE YOURSELF WHEN YOU DESERVE IT

TRUST YOUR OWN JUDGMENT

LOVE YOURSELF

The next page is a cognitive therapy worksheet. When I had cognitive therapy at the University of Pennsylvania clinic, the patient had a specific number of sessions. In my case, that meant 10. To the best of my knowledge this type of treatment was discovered and refined by Dr. Aaron Beck and Dr. David Burns. In fact, a book was published entitled *Feeling Good*. The basic concept involves understanding and controlling automatic thoughts that is a category listed on the third column of the worksheet.

YOU CAN IMPROVE YOUR SELF-ESTEEM. IT'S REALLY WORTH THE EFFORT THOUGH IT'S HARD WORK.

Date	Situation / Event Describe 1. Actual event leading to unpleasant emotion, or 2. Stream of thoughts, day-dream, or recollection leading to unpleasant emotion	Emotions 1. specify and anxious / angry etc. 2. Rate degree of emotion 1 - 100	Automatic Thoughts 1. Write automatic thought(s) that preceded emotion(s) 2. Rate belief in automatic thought(s) 0 - 100	Rational Response 1. Write rational response in automatic thought(s) 2. Rate belief in rational response. 0 - 100	Outcome 1. Rerate belief in automatic thought(s). 0 - 100 2. Specify and rate subsequent emotions. 0 - 100

Instructions: When you experience an unpleasant emotion, note the situation that seemed to stimulate the emotion. (If the emotion occurred while you were thinking, daydreaming, etc. please note this.)   Then note the automatic thought associated with the emotion. Record the degree to which you believe this thought: 0 = not at all, 100 = completely. In rating degree of emotion 1 = a trace; 100 = the most intense possible.

As my self-esteem grew and I continued my leadership of self-help groups, I realized I could make a difference in the future of mental health treatment. But I never dreamed that I could be a strategic part of a movement that would shift the treatment of patients to those who themselves had experienced the hopelessness and desperation that are the hallmarks of being mentally ill.

The closing of Byberry, the Philadelphia State Hospital, with its long cycle of abuse, neglect and inadequate care, became my goal along with that of numerous mental health organizations and individuals. Those of us who have been locked up in places like this know the importance of treatment that will return us to the community where we can be productive, develop meaningful relationships and fulfill our lives.

Our goal was to replace Byberry with a humane system of care defined by consumer-run programs for former Byberry residents—drop-in centers, housing, self-help, advocacy, vocational education and social support services. We believed that mental health consumers, especially those who have experienced institutionalization, were uniquely skilled in understanding and meeting the needs of their peers. They could provide safer and more effective services for those who needed them. In addition, instead of depending on disability benefits or other entitlements for support, they could become self-sufficient.

The advocacy movement was astonishingly successful. The closing of Byberry opened the door to a community system of mental health services. People who used to live there moved into structured residences. Some went to work. Some went to day programs. They made friends. The changes in them were remarkable. In my dark days, I never could have imagined that I would play a significant role in this dramatic shift in mental health treatment. We called it the Byberry Miracle.

Five years later, I became a founding member of Advocates for the Jewish Mentally Ill: Tikvah (which means hope) spearheaded as a social organization by Judy Schulman Zon, a woman whose son Rlichard who suffered, as I did, from bipolar illness. It was the first such organization in the Jewish community, although you didn't need to be Jewish to join. We started meeting at Judy's home, and little by little through word of mouth, the organization grew. Two leading psychiatrists, Paul Fink and Lawrence Real, were our advisors.

Lucky for us, incredible Mike Sloane who was concerned, as many of our members were, about housing for those with mental illness, found and purchased a small apartment house in the Philadelphia suburbs open to Tikvah members. It was filled quickly, and over the years the demand continued to be high. Today there is a waiting list.

Tikvah morphed from a small volunteer-run group to one that now has professional status. Its office space is donated by the Federation of Jewish Agencies and there is a part-time executive director. Tikvah's mission has moved toward increasing opportunities for much needed social interaction among those with mental illness, producing a monthly calendar crammed with events—dinners, lectures, bowling outings, Bingo parties. The goal is to reduce isolation and increase independence for those who are mentally ill. Each year, I present an award in my parents' name to someone who has given exemplary service to the cause of mental illness. I am proud to be Tikvah's co-president. But there are people out there we're still not reaching. And they need us. We have to keep spreading the message. Self-help is powerful in developing relationships, friendships and providing support for each other in a safe social haven. A former president of the group had her first birthday party when she was 40. She said that she used to feel isolated, without friends, with nowhere to go. Mostly, she would not leave her bed. Since joining Tikvah, she has cherished relationships and a reason to get up every day.

Alison Malmon was a student at the University of Pennsylvania when her older brother committed suicide. To fight campus stigma of mental illness and to encourage those students who suffer from it to seek help early, she developed Open Minds. It is a student group with the mission of helping every young person understand and empathize with those who are mentally ill. I worked with Alison to get her program started. Since then, she has developed chapters of what is now called Active Minds on college campuses throughout the country because she knows how vulnerable college students are to mental disorders. Headquarters are in Washington DC.

We need more attention to young people with mental illness because the statistics are staggering:

- 27% of young adults between 18-24 have the highest prevalence of diagnosable mental illness
- Half of all adults with depression report onset before age 20
- Bipolar disorder typically develops in late adolescence or early adulthood; so does schizophrenia
- Suicide is the third leading cause of death among those 18-24, and the second leading cause of death for college students. 95% of those suffer from a mental illness

As former Surgeon General David Satcher recognized almost two decades ago, "Mental disorders are real illnesses that are as disabling and serious as cancer and heart disease in terms of premature death and lost productivity. Few Americans are untouched by it whether it occurs within one's family or among neighbors, co-workers or members of the community."

Now that I am stable and productive, it is my pledge to spend the rest of my life making a difference in the lives of people who are in the place I was for so long.

Epilogue

After many years, this final version of my book, which began as a diary during an inpatient stay at Bryn Mawr Hospital's Psychiatric Unit, has been put to bed. It has taken a great deal of effort to produce this manuscript, and its completion is testimony to how someone with extreme bipolar disorder can come full circle and bring a message of healing and hope to others.

For those of you living with a mental illness, I urge you to "come out of the closet" and speak honestly with an open heart. Just remember that these conditions are only a small part of who you are. Keep in mind that relationships require work to be successful. That pertains to family, friends and especially with a romantic partner. If you fall in love with someone and continue to hide your illness, stress will inevitably develop which will leave you more vulnerable to emotional pain.

If you are a family member, remember to be patient, as difficult as it sometimes is. Your loved one has the capacity to achieve a sense of well-being. Don't lose hope. Remember to take care of yourself and keep reminding yourself that it's not your fault that your child, sibling, parent or spouse is dealing with a mental illness. We all need to learn from each other. That includes psychiatrists, psychologists and all therapists. While your patient must be your first priority, it is critical to keep the family involved during treatment. A mentally ill person can't have enough support during his or her struggle for wellness.

I continue to speak publicly to educate others. Continue to gain strength from spirituality and read a portion of the Old Testament every week. My wife, Judy, deserves all the love and consideration I can give her. Acts of kindness, charity and prayer are important components of my life. Hopefully, my friendships will keep growing. I recognize that surrounding myself with healthy, positive people will go a long way toward maintaining my recovery and stability.

64

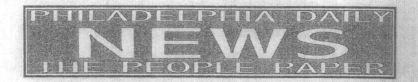

Opinion

A TALE OF TWO MIKES

Mentally Ill Need Someone in Their Corner

"Now I have two things in common with the heavyweight champion. We're both named Mike, and we're both manic depressives."

Mike Solomon is considering that line as an opener to the speech he's giving this week in Cleveland. After a panel discussion at Temple University Hospital Monday, he's going on the road, trying to spread a little more understanding of his sickness.

Mike Solomon has followed the soap opera-like sagas of the unhappy heavyweight champ with empathy and concern, as the ominous, vulnerable Mike Tyson and his manipulative wife, Robin Givens, have played out the pathetic days of their lives for all to see.

From Solomon's point of view, the "Mike and Robin Show" is sad and bad news. Rather than enhancing public understanding of mental illness, it feeds all the usual stereotypes.

Solomon, diagnosed as manic-depressive at 19, is 34. He's lived a full and relatively stable life, thanks to a supportive mother and a dad who always kept a place for Mike in his business.

He has a bachelor's degree from Villanova and is now enrolled in graduate school there, with plans to become a counselor. He's also a volunteer coordinator for support groups for manic depressives, and supported by the Philadelphia Psychiatric Center (now called Belmont Hospital). He knows what he'd say if he had Mike Tyson's ear.

First, he'd try to get a sense of how Tyson really feels, so he'd stop denying his problems.

"I'd ask him, when you smashed that car, were you really feeling suicidal, like you wanted to die? And when you punched that guy, why did you really do it?"

I can't say he's manic-depressive, but I'd say, "Mike, you're 22, and this usually hits young adults." And I'd urge him to shop around until he can find a doctor he can relate to even if it means going to 10.

Reports this week indicate that Tyson went to a new doctor, who declared that he's not manic-depressive, as his wife has contended and he has denied.

Solomon is skeptical: "I'd tell Tyson to forget about liking what doctors tell you and find someone you can work with."

Solomon admits that lithium, drug of choice for treatment of manic depressives, does have some side effects including blurred vision, excessive thirst, and "slowing you down" an athlete's nightmare. It is the medication Tyson reportedly stopped taking because it made him feel "bad."

Lithium is toxic. Monthly blood tests are required to maintain proper balance, and an overdose can kill.

Controlling the illness is the centerpiece of every manic depressive's life. Trying to coordinate psychotherapy and medication to cope with the devastating lows, when suicidal tendencies emerge, and the giddy (or irritable) highs, Solomon's problem and maybe Tyson's camouflaged by the "outlet" of boxing.

What troubles Solomon is that Tyson is a boxer, a man who is violent for a living and in his free time, breaking furniture, driving into trees, punching sparring partners and allegedly roughing up his wife. All of that exacerbates the misconceptions about mental illness that Solomon and others want to dispel.

"I've never hit anybody," says Solomon, "even when I was in bad shape." Statistics indicate that the mentally ill are no more violent than the general population.

Solomon points out that in spite of care in taking lithium, he gets sick often enough to be hospitalized, usually when he slips into a "high" or manic phase. His actions at such times take the form of intense exuberance. Once he was on the phone with a friend late at night, and he decided to drive over for a visit all the way to North Carolina. He was pulled over in Washington D.C., falling asleep at the wheel. Another time, he took off on a spree to Atlantic City, gambling, tipping big, and romping wildly on the beach.

Though he perhaps would prefer another metaphor, Solomon is a fighter, a tough guy who refused to give in to a difficult and much misunderstood disease. Through medication and therapy and perseverance, he's always bounced back. His marriage failed, and his dad is dead now but he's still determined to have an independent life.

"The best thing you can do is not to give in. Don't sleep all day long," he says. "There's lots of research being done, support groups, and there's hope."

After patients accept their illness and learn to cope, the biggest issue is acceptance by others, being able to say "I am sick," and having people be supportive.

"It's not what people will say, it's what they won't say, and how they act," Solomon said. "People you thought were friends, you don't hear from them."

In all his hospitalizations, Mike says, he's never gotten a card, a letter or a phone call from members of his family, other than his parents.

"That's rough," he says simply. "If things were reversed, I know I'd be there for them."

Ultimately, illness and wellness do not alter human needs for what we all want, but sometimes, like Mike Tyson, can't find someone to be in our corner, to share and to care about us.

For general information on mental illness, contact the Mental Health Association of Southeastern Pennsylvania at (215) 751-1800

Linda Wright Moore's column appears on Fridays.

About the Authors:

Michael Solomon:

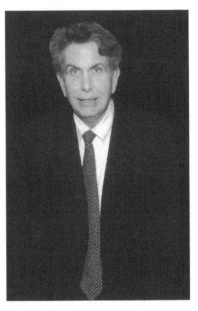

Michael has lived with Bipolar Illness since the summer of 1974. However, the initial diagnosis was Depression. In 1975 at the Carrier Clinic/Foundation, doctors changed Michael's diagnosis to Bipolar which started him on a journey into the world of Mental Health/Illness.

Since that time and despite many mood swings and challenges that accompany Bipolar Illness, Michael has worked primarily in the helping profession.

A one-time sales manager for AMS Brokerage (Abraham Martin Solomon)—a father and son food brokerage business, Michael lives in Montgomery County, PA with his wife Judy, a retired school teacher, and their three television sets.

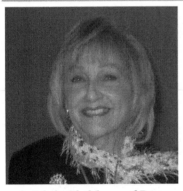

Gloria Hochman:

Gloria Hochman is a New York Times best-selling author and has won 23 journalism awards for her article writing in health, psychology and social issues. Her books include: *A Brilliant Madness: Living with Manic-Depressive Illness* which she co-authored with the late actor Patty Duke. Her other books are *Heart Bypass: What Every Patient Must Know* and *Adult Children of Divorce* which she co-authored with Washington DC psychiatrist Edward W. Beal. She was editor and wrote several chapters for the e-book, *The Age for Change*, published by Temple University's Intergenerational Center, AARP, Pennsylvania and the United Way of Southeastern Pennsylvania. It explores issues facing baby boomers as they re-brand the vision of aging.

Ms. Hochman has published hundred of articles for The Philadelphia Inquirer where she writes for the newspaper's health and science section, Newsweek, Psychology Today, Reader's Digest and Science Digest. She has reviewed books for the New York Times.

For more than 25 years, she has directed communications for the Philadelphia-based National Adoption Center where she is responsible for media relations, writes and edits the Center's print and online publications, moderates public forums on adoption and child welfare issues, and works closely with the executive director to carry out the Center's mission.

Gloria Hochman
Gloriahochman.com
215-588-0506
gloriahoch@comcast.net

Do Not Quit

When things go wrong as they sometimes will…
When the road you're trudging seems all up hill…
When the funds are low and the debts are high…
And you want to smile, but you have to sigh…
When care is pressing you down a bit…
Rest if you must, but don't you quit.

Life is queer with its twists and turns
As everyone of us sometimes learns
And many a person turns about

When they might have won had they stuck it out
Don't give up though the pace seems slow
You may succeed with another blow
Often the struggler has given up
When he might have captured the victor's cup
And he learned too late when the night came down
How close he was to the golden crown
Success is failure turned inside out
So stick to the fight when you're hardest hit
It's when things seem worst that you must NOT
QUIT

Copyright by Violet Bowers

10963888R00044

Made in the USA
Lexington, KY
08 October 2018